Coconut Oil

100 Plus Uses for Coconut Oil!

Learn all the Amazing Health Benefits and the Many Secrets for Coconut Oil

(Secret Coconut Oil Recipes Included!)

Table of Contents

Introduction

I want to thank you and congratulate you for downloading the book, *"100 plus uses for Coconut Oil! Learn all the Amazing Health Benefits and the Many Secrets for Coconut Oil. (Secret Coconut Oil Recipes Included!)"*.

This book contains proven steps and strategies on how to use coconut oil in improving your health and giving yourself a better appearance. Inside are 100+ uses for coconut oil, as well as instructions on how you can create homemade items from it.

There was never a doubt that coconut oil is indeed a miracle product. Its uses are pretty diverse – some include boosting brains of Alzheimer's patients, reduces wrinkles and cellulites, and helps in losing weight. Other uses include functioning as a homemade mascara, eye liner, lipstick, and many more.

It is a product that has uses for your head down to your toe. You can use it even on your household items and on your pets. Its endless benefits make it one of the best products to have inside your pantry.

Inside this book are a couple of recipes you can try at home, with ingredients so simple that you do not have to go far to get them. Most of all, you will get to know the many benefits that you will enjoy in the long run.

Thanks again for downloading this book, I hope you enjoy it!

Chapter 1
The Wonders of Coconut Oil

Coconut oil is one of the most useful substances there is – the ways on how you can use it are virtually endless. There are a lot of ways on how you can use it, and you get many benefits out of it.

How many ways can you use coconut oil? Literally hundreds of ways. Or maybe thousands. That is why it is called a "superfood". You would be able to find a use for it for your head to toe. There are uses as well that will fit all ages; coconut oil will benefit babies and adults alike.

The Good Oil that is Coconut Oil

What is good about coconut oil? It is a natural oil that is antifungal, antibacterial, and anti-inflammatory. It may even help fight cancer. A lot of infections can be alleviated by coconut oil, and can even fight parasites such as tapeworms and lice. It does a lot without making you experience any awful side effects.

There are two kinds of coconut oil: refined and unrefined.

a. **Refined coconut oil** is also called "expeller pressed". You know it is coconut oil, but it does not taste or smell like coconut oil. The process it undergoes takes out some of its nutrition, so while it still functions the same, it is not as nutritious and effective.

b. **Unrefined coconut oil** is more popularly known as the "virgin" or "extra virgin" coconut oil. It is in its natural state and has not undergone any major processes. If you use it for cooking, you will get a bit of coconut flavor. Applying it externally will also give you hints of coconut. All nutrition remains on the unrefined coconut oil, so it is more effective compared to refined coconut oil.

Benefits of Coconut Oil

Coconut oil's unique blend of fatty acids make it one of the most beneficial substances. Its benefits include better brain function, fat loss, and other amazing benefits.

Trying to name all coconut oil benefits will be impossible, so here is just a few of them to give you an idea of the awesomeness of coconut oil.

Coconut oil has strong medicinal properties

People used to shun coconut oil because of the saturated fat you can get from it. However, studies prove that the saturated fat in coconut oil will not harm you because its fats actually contain MCTs or Medium Chain Triglycerides.

What is good about MCTs? MCTs are built differently from the usual saturated fats; they are of medium length, which means they are metabolized differently. From your digestive tract, MCTs go straight to your liver and get transformed to either an energy source, or ketone bodies that can give therapeutic effects on various brain disorders such as Alzheimer's and epilepsy.

Coconut oil helps you burn more amounts of fat by increasing your energy expenditure

Weight gain and obesity is often connected to calories, yet have you ever considered that it's not just about the calories, but also where you're getting the calories from?

Foods affect your body in different ways, and the food's effect on you will depend on the kind of food you are eating. If the food brings you positive effects, then the calories you get from it most likely will bring positive effects, too.

Again, the MCTs are responsible for this. MCTs help increase energy expenditure by 5%, which is equal to about 120 calories each day. This additional energy consumption will potentially lead to a significant weight loss in the long run.

Coconut oil can stop you from feeling hungry

Yes, coconut oil can actually lessen your hunger. As previously mentioned, coconut oil has ketone bodies, and these ketone bodies help reduce your appetite.

A study was in fact done to six men, and they were asked to take coconut oil with MCTs. After a while, it was observed that these men ate, on average, 256 fewer calories each day. Plus, an intake of MCT during breakfast would also decrease their calorie intake come lunch time.

Prolonged instances of fewer calorie intake will lead to weight loss; better results will be achieved if coupled with exercise.

Coconut oil is good for the heart

The saturated fats found in coconut oil do not harm the heart. What they do is raise the body's HDL (good cholesterol) and change LDL (harmful cholesterol) to a less destructive form.

Coconut oil reduces the body's triglycerides, LDL and total cholesterol levels while increasing HDL and improving the body's antioxidant status and blood coagulation factors. This leads to less chances of acquiring or developing heart diseases.

Coconut oil helps eliminate bacteria, fungi and viruses

Coconut oil, once digested, also forms monolaurin, a monoglyceride that helps kill pathogens such as bacteria, fungi and viruses. Coconut oil also has lauric acid that functions the same as monolaurin.

Both substances can help kill Staphylococcus aureus and Candida albicans, dangerous elements that cause harm to humans.

Coconut oil intake not only helps kill harmful pathogens but also help prevent infections, making you stronger.

Coconut oil helps boost brains of patients afflicted by Alzheimer's

There are elderly individuals who get inflicted with Alzheimer's disease. Having Alzheimer's disease means your body finds it harder to use glucose and convert it to energy for certain parts of the brain.

Ketone bodies can provide energy to the brain; according to researchers, ketones can possibly provide an alternate source of energy to the malfunctioning cells and lessen Alzheimer's symptoms.

Those are just few of the benefits you can get from coconut oil. The following chapters will state how you can use coconut oil in different ways, as well as share additional benefits that you can take advantage of.

Chapter 2
Uses for Coconut Oil: Beauty

Beauty products nowadays come in different chemicals that you know nothing about. Why not use coconut oil instead? Did you know that coconut oil can substitute for most of the items in your make-up kit?

Concerned for your skin (especially that of your face)? Read on to know how you can use coconut oil to give yourself that healthier glow.

1. You can put a little amount on a cotton ball and use coconut oil to remove eye makeup. It leaves the under eye area hydrated as well.

2. It also functions as a moisturizer when you rub the oil all over your face and neck. Just wash the residue off using your favorite cleanser.

3. Mix coconut oil with salt or brown sugar to make an effective body scrub.

4. Coconut oil can be used as a massage oil. It is skin-friendly and slippery. It moisturizes while alleviating your sore muscles.

5. Sweeping a small amount of coconut oil on top of your makeup can serve as a highlighter for your cheekbones.

6. You can use coconut oil for your own homemade lip balm that helps get rid of dry and cracked lips.

7. Coconut oil also helps reduce wrinkles and helps prevent premature aging. For better results, mix coconut oil with frankincense oil.

8. You can use coconut oil to make your own homemade mascara.

9. Coconut oil can also be used as an ingredient for your homemade eye liner; just mix 2 teaspoons of coconut oil with aloe vera gel, together with either ½ teaspoon of cocoa powder (for brown) or activated charcoal (for black). Store the mixture in an airtight container.

10. Oily stuff trigger acne, right? But in this case, coconut oil helps prevent acne. Acne is caused by both greasy and dry skin – in

this case, coconut oil helps moisturize dry skin, hence preventing acne breakouts.

11. Coconut oil removes the puffiness around your eyes. To have a fresh and youthful appearance, dab a few drops of coconut oil around your eyes prior to sleeping. You will see a less puffy appearance upon waking up in the morning.

12. You can mix coconut oil and castor oil together to have a deep cleansing and effective face wash.

13. Not only can coconut oil be used as a shaving cream, but also as an aftershave. Using coconut oil will soothe irritation and reduces the chance of you getting razor burn.

14. Mixing coconut oil with baking soda will produce a good exfoliating agent that helps remove both dead skin cells and dirt from your face. You will see results when you are done.

15. Applying coconut oil to your age spots will help them fade faster. Applying them regularly will give you the best results.

16. You can use coconut oil to exfoliate your lips. By mixing coconut oil with brown sugar and honey (optional), you will have a mixture that will be able to exfoliate your lips but not damage them.

17. Applying a drop or two of coconut oil directly on your lips will help keep them moist and healthy.

18. Mixing honey and coconut oil will produce a homemade face mask. Mix them until you achieve a consistency similar to that of the usual face masks. Just apply it to your skin, wait for about fifteen minutes, and then wash your face. Your complexion will be clearer and will have a nice glow.

19. Coconut oil can help shield your face and skin with its SPF 4 protection. Mix it with aloe vera gel to achieve a better combination. Don't stay out on the sun too long, though, as this only provides basic protection.

20. The lauric acid found in coconut oil can help treat cold sores. All you need is to mix 5 drops of oregano with 2 tablespoons of coconut oil, and apply this mixture on the cold sore instantly when you see it.

Chapter 3
Uses of Coconut Oil: Skin & Hair

It is not enough that you have great skin on your face – the benefits should be shown in the whole body, as well as the hair.

Coconut oil is ideal for hair and skin care because it works as an effective moisturizer. It is also recommended because it does not pose any negative side effects on the skin.

Have healthier skin and hair through the help of coconut oil.

21. You can put a little oil to soothe your dry hands. It can also be used instead of your usual body lotion. Focus on dry and rough spots such as knees and elbows.

22. You can use it as an antimicrobial and inexpensive shaving cream that hydrates your legs. It will also help in preventing growth of ingrown hairs and even lessen chances of razor burn.

23. You can use it as a conditioner that penetrates hair better; apply a quarter-

sized amount, comb your hair, and pull your hair to a loose bun. You can either place a soft towel on your pillow or use a shower cap. Shampoo your hair the next morning.

24. Adding coconut oil at the ends of your hair can help add a little shine. It also helps tame flyaways especially if your hair is darker. Be careful though; too much coconut oil will make your hair look and feel greasy.

25. Rubbing coconut oil onto your cuticles will help repel germs; it will also help loosen up your cuticles and make it easier for you to cut or push them back.

26. Babies will also love coconut oil because it helps ease the redness, itch, and pain of diaper rash. Simply use a tablespoon over the affected area.

27. Use coconut oil on your hair and scalp to moisturize the area and prevent dandruff growth.

28. Coconut oil also works for skin conditions such as psoriasis and eczema.

29. Coconut oil helps reduce visibility of stretch marks – it makes them fade more quickly while moisturizing your skin.

30. It can help reduce skin redness, rehydrate and soothe inflamed skin caused by sunburn. Adding zinc oxide or red raspberry seed extract will make your homemade sunblock stronger.

31. You can mix ylang ylang oil with coconut oil and anise oil to create a spray that is effective in treating head lice, especially for children.

32. Placing coconut oil on your eyelashes will help make them grow longer.

33. Mixing coconut oil with a bit of sea salt will create a coarse exfoliating mixture that will work great for your feet. This is also a way of softening hard soles.

34. You can also get rid of cellulite through coconut oil. First, do dry brushing i.e. sweep a soft-bristled brush upwards toward the heart, and then follow up with coconut oil on the same areas. After regular application, you will notice reduced cellulite marks.

35. Coconut oil can help treat canker sores. Just use a cotton swab to apply coconut oil directly onto the canker sore. The coconut oil will then fight infections that led to the canker sore and speed up the healing process.

36. You can use coconut oil to reduce the appearance of varicose veins. Just apply it directly as a topical ointment regularly to see the best results.

37. You can remove babies' cradle caps using coconut oil – you just have to massage the oil onto the baby's head, then leave on for a couple of minutes. Rinse it off after using a warm wash cloth.

38. Bruises will heal faster and their swelling will be reduced by placing coconut oil on them.

39. After getting a tattoo, coconut oil can serve as an effective moisturizer. The oil speeds up the tattoo's healing process and even lessens the tattoo's chances of infection. Don't overdo it, though, as applying too much coconut oil can bleach the ink and reduce the color's brightness.

40. Coconut oil can be used for oil pulling; what you do is swish an amount of coconut oil inside your mouth for about 20 minutes a day prior to brushing your teeth. Once you are done, spit in the trash and not the sink because coconut oil can end up clogging the drains.

Chapter 4
Uses of Coconut Oil: Food

Just thinking of your favorite food can make you happy; what more if you are going to incorporate coconut oil into them, making them healthier?

Here are some ways on how you can use coconut oil for your food.

41. You can use cooking oil for frying and sautéing. It has a high smoke point that is why it is ideal for cooking in high heat. Its healthy saturated fats still stay stable even at high temperatures.

42. Coconut oil can be used as a coffee creamer. Blend hot coffee with coconut oil and you will instantly have a natural sweetener that is rich and creamy sans the additional dairy.

43. Adding a tablespoon or two to your usual fruit smoothies will add more cholesterol fighting compounds. Better yet, your smoothies have improved texture and mouth feel.

44. The eggs in your fridge will have a longer shelf life, thanks to coconut oil. What you

do is swipe a little bit of oil over the eggs' shells and leave it for a while for the oil to penetrate. Eggs will now last longer for about 1-2 weeks.

45. Coconut oil can serve as an alternative for a healthier mayonnaise. In a blender, mix one tablespoon of apple cider vinegar, 4 egg yolks and dried mustard. Mix until all ingredients are combined. As the blender runs, add the cup of melted coconut oil, slowly, as well as half a cup of olive oil to have an emulsion.

Note: The mayo will break if you add the oils hastily. In this case, don't worry, just add tahini, about a tablespoon, and blend them until smooth.

46. Instead of butter, coconut oil can also be used as a popcorn topping.

47. Coconut oil can also be used as a salad dressing.

48. Coconut oil can serve as a substitute not only for butter but also for vegetable oils and margarine for baking.

49. You can use coconut oil to bake homemade granola bars and will give a "coconutty" scent to oats and nuts.

50. Coconut oil can be mixed into a mug of hot cocoa.

51. Coconut oil can also be used whenever you are roasting vegetables. Just mix coconut oil with lemon juice, salt, pepper and thyme or rosemary, and toss the vegetables with this mixture.

52. You can use coconut oil as an ingredient for cupcake frostings. *

53. You can rub chicken with seasonings and coconut oil prior to roasting.

54. Coconut oil can be used as an ingredient for ice cream. *

55. You can create your homemade peanut butter by grinding 2 cups of peanuts (or you can substitute them with cashews, almonds or pecans) with 2 tablespoons of coconut oil. You can even add honey, cinnamon, maple syrup or flaxseed for a more unique blend.

*-Recipe found in a later chapter

Chapter 5
Uses of Coconut Oil: Brain & Body

In the previous chapters, coconut oil gave you a prettier face and a happier tummy. Why not make yourself completely healthier? And smarter?

Here are uses of coconut oil that will benefit both your brain and your body.

56. Because of its antifungal properties, coconut oil can help fight athlete's foot. Just rub a few drops of coconut oil on your foot several instances a day.

57. Coconut oil can also be used to make homemade toothpaste. You can mix coconut oil and baking soda plus a couple of drops of peppermint essential oil. You can also add stevia to make it a little bit sweeter.

58. Stubborn cellulite can be fought using coconut oil. Mix a tablespoon of coconut oil with about 10 drops of grapefruit

essential oil. Massage into affected areas in firm, circular motions.

59. Your dry and cracked heels will soon find relief with coconut oil. Rub them with coconut oil and allow the oil to be absorbed by your skin. You can mix coconut oil with other essential oils such as lavender oil to help lessen dryness and bacteria, plus give your feet a nice and relaxing scent.

60. You can use coconut oil as a topical ointment that helps relieve the pain brought by hemorrhoids.

61. Coconut oil has soothing properties that can help provide relief from the irritation and itch brought by chicken pox. What you do is add coconut oil in your warm bath with oatmeal, and soak on it.

62. You can use coconut oil to treat hay fever. All you do is dab a bit of coconut oil in every nostril. It works by having the pollen and other allergens stick to the oil instead of getting into your nose.

63. Instead of Lanolin cream, you can use coconut oil to soothe irritated nursing nipples.

64. Studies show that regular intake of coconut oil can help avoid or prevent Alzheimer's disease.

65. Drinking hot tea with a tablespoon of coconut oil can help speed up your recovery from colds or flu.

66. A part of coconut oil mixed with two parts of clove oil will help provide fast relief for toothache. Just use cotton balls or swabs to apply this mixture gently on the affected tooth.

67. Coconut oil can also help you when you have colds. Mix coconut oil with eucalyptus oil for a natural vapor rub that relieves the discomfort brought by colds. Just rub the blend on your chest to open up clogged airways and have better breathing.

68. You can use it as an ingredient for a homemade cough syrup. Just mix 3 tablespoons of lemon juice with 2 tablespoons of coconut oil and ¼ cup of raw honey. Place the mixture over low heat until your coconut oil is melted. To take it, you can either mix it on water or tea, or take a mixture by the spoonful.

69. Coconut oil helps you lose weight. Aside from serving as a healthy alternative to certain ingredients, taking two tablespoons of coconut oil a day will help speed up your metabolism, leading to weight loss.

70. Coconut oil can also help you improve your digestion.

71. You will get a good night sleep through the use of coconut oil. Coconut oil can be mixed with essential oils such as lavender oil to help fight anxiety, calm the min, and have better, quality sleep.

72. Coconut oil can help alleviate the pain caused by bee stings, as well as skin infected by oak, sumac or poison ivy. All you need is apply coconut oil directly on the affected area.

73. Research shows that massaging newborn babies with coconut oil can help promote growth and weight gain.

74. Coconut oil can also be used in aromatherapy. Its soothing scent can be pleasing, and it can help you relax after a long and stressful day.

75. A teaspoon of coconut oil is said to better energize you than a cup of coffee or a bottle of energy drink.

76. You can use coconut oil to treat yeast infections because of its caprylic acid and lauric acid; the fatty acids in coconut oil is said to help kill candida found in the intestines.

77. Coconut oil is also said to help relieve and treat heartburn or acid reflux as it soothes your esophagus.

78. By swirling a mixture of honey and coconut oil and then swallowing the said mixture, you will be relieved of the pains of sore throat. As it travels down your throat, it will be soothed and you will soon feel better.

79. Coconut oil helps prevent nose bleeding. Nose that gets dry easily, hence frequent nose bleeds, can be prevented by placing a bit of coconut oil in the area and moisturizing the nostrils. By doing so, your nasal passages won't dry out.

80. Taking three tablespoons of coconut oil will help treat urinary tract infection (UTI)

because of the coconut oil's antimicrobial properties.

Chapter 6
Uses of Coconut Oil: Pets & Household

Want more reasons to love coconut oil? Well, it is not only good for you, but also good for your pets! Yes, coconut oil can also be used for your beloved animals on which your fur babies get to experience the benefits.

Here are some ways on how you can use coconut oil for your pets and home:

81. It can be used as a topical ointment that promotes the healing of wounds, bites, cuts, stings and hot spots. Coconut oil is edible, so your pets won't have problems if they end up licking it.

82. Placing coconut oil on your cat's paws can promote a shiny coat plus lessen chances of hairballs.

83. Coconut oil can also help soothe a dog's dry nose.

84. The intake of coconut oil can give a dog a shiny coat.

85. Pets with upset tummies can take one to two teaspoons of coconut oil mixed with their food.

86. Taking coconut oil will also help deodorize doggy scent.

87. Coconut oil can serve as a shoe shiner; all you need to do is use coconut oil on your patent heels or leather boots to hide their blemishes, make them shiny, and make them look like new all over again.

88. Stuck zippers? You can just apply a few drops of coconut oil and wait a few moments to get them unstuck.

89. Coconut oil can also be mixed to olive oil to become a homemade laundry soap.

90. Got rust on metal items inside the household? Rub coconut oil on your outdoor metal furniture, silverware, car parts, or other metal items that need polishing. It helps remove rust when you place a thin layer over the metal item for 1-2 hours. You can choose to simply wipe off the oil or wash the item completely. You will see results right away.

91. You can mix coconut oil with rosemary, mint, or even catnip as a natural repellent for bugs.

92. Coconut oil can serve as a lubricant for different electronic items and even in small motors.

93. You can use coconut oil to remove caked-on foods from your dishes, instead of placing more dishwashing pastes or elbow grease on them. These tough spots will then be softer, and washing will be a breeze.

94. Coconut oil helps keep your shower squeaky clean. Instead of using harsh chemicals, you can just use a rag with coconut oil and remove shower scum. You will be done in no time.

95. You can use coconut oil to make your own homemade insect repellent. Eight ounces of coconut oil can be mixed with about 40-50 drops of essential oil such as eucalyptus, lemongrass, mint, clove and citronella. Reapply throughout the day to maximize protection.

96. Coconut oil can be used to remove hardened gum residue. It works on pretty

much any surface, even in hair, and on your carpets.

97. Do you own a guitar? You can also use coconut oil to condition and lubricate your guitar strings.

98. Coconut oil can also be used to remove all the clumps and buildup on your mascara brush. All you need to do is soak your mascara brush in about five minutes. If there are any remaining clumps, your fingers can just easily remove them.

99. Do not get creeped at night – use coconut oil to lubricate any squeaky hinges in your home. Just apply a few drops of coconut oil to the squeaky hinge to lubricate it and stop it from squeaking.

100. Starting a campfire? Do not use lighter fluid – use coconut oil. All you need to do is soak cotton balls with them and light them up. With dried twigs and leaves, you've got a good campfire going.

Chapter 6
Coconut Oil Recipes

One of the main purposes of coconut oil is to serve as an ingredient for different recipes. The recipes you can use coconut oil vary from foods to beauty creams and to various household items, proving how useful and versatile coconut oil is.

See how amazing your recipes will be with coconut oil. Try these simple recipes out, and once you've tried their finished products, you'll decide never to run out of coconut oil again.

Peach Yogurt Muffins

Ingredients:

- Sugar, ¾ cup
- All-purpose flour, 2 cups
- Baking powder, ½ teaspoon
- Baking soda, ½ teaspoon
- Salt, ½ teaspoon
- Eggs, 2
- Plain Greek yogurt, 1 cup
- Nonfat milk, 1 cup
- Coconut oil, melted, ¼ cup plus 2 teaspoons
- Fresh or frozen peaches, chopped, 1 ½ cup

Instructions:

Grease your large muffin pan as you preheat the oven to 350°F.

In a large bowl, combine and whisk together sugar, flour, baking soda, baking powder, salt and cinnamon. In a separate bowl, whisk eggs, coconut oil, greek yogurt and milk.

Pour the wet ingredients immediately into the dry ingredients together with the chopped peaches; mix together using a spatula until combined. Don't overmix.

Scoop batter into your muffin pan. Bake the muffins for about 20-23 minutes. Cool them in pan for about 5 minutes, and then transfer them gently to a cooling rack.

Coconut Crusted Mahi Mahi Nuggets

Ingredients:

- Mahi Mahi, 1 ¼ lb.
- Almond flour, 1 cup
- Egg, large, 1
- Extra virgin coconut oil, ¼ cup
- Unsweetened coconut, finely shredded, 2/3 cup
- Salt, ¾ tsp
- Pepper, ¼ tsp
- Lime wedges, 4

Instructions:

Prepare a wire rack for cooling placed over the cookie sheet you're about to use. Set aside.

Cut your mahi mahi to your preferred size, usually about an inch or two. Pat them dry using your paper towels.

Whisk the egg inside a large bowl. Combine coconut, almond flour, pepper and salt in a plastic container. Place on lid, secure, and shake the container to mix all ingredients.

In a large skillet, heat over medium heat around 2 tbsp. of your coconut oil. Add ½ of the mahi

mahi to the whisked egg. Toss them both to coat. Transfer coated pieces to your mixture with almond flour using forks or slotted spoons, shaking off the excess egg.

Place the lid on your container; shake until all fish pieces are coated well. Move the pieces of fish to the skillet and then cook each side for about 2-4 minutes, or until light golden brown.

Transfer cooked pieces to wire rack. Repeat with the rest of the fish.

Serve the fish pieces with your lime wedges.

Vinegar and Coco Oil Salad Dressing

Ingredients:

- Coconut oil, ¼ cup
- Raw honey, ½ teaspoon
- Vinegar, 1 tablespoon
- Himalayan Salt, ¼ teaspoon

Instructions:

Combine coconut oil and vinegar in a small metal bowl. Whisk briskly until thick. Add honey, then salt. Whisk until the mixture is well combined.

To thin the mixture, place the bowl in a saucepan with simmering water. Continue stirring the mixture. It'll soon be liquefied and will be ready once it reaches room temperature.

Sweet Potatoes Roasted in Coconut Oil

Ingredients:

- Coconut oil, 2 tablespoons
- Ground black pepper, ¼ teaspoon
- Grated lime zest, 1 teaspoon
- Sweet potatoes, 2 pounds, cut in 1-inch chunks
- Fine sea salt, ½ teaspoon

Instructions:

Preheat the oven to 400°F. Melt the coconut oil in a saucepan over medium heat. Toss the potatoes with salt, pepper and oil in a large bowl until the potatoes are evenly coated.

Spread the potatoes on a large baking sheet in a single layer. Roast potatoes for about 40 minutes or until tender. Transfer potatoes in a serving bowl; toss potatoes with lime zest.

Coco Cupcake Frosting

Ingredients:

- Coconut oil, 1 ¼ cup
- Honey or agave nectar, 1 cup
- Water, 1 tablespoon
- Celtic sea salt, a pinch
- Arrowroot powder, 5 teaspoons
- Coconut milk, 1 cup

Instructions:

Heat honey, coconut milk and salt in a saucepan and simmer for about 10 minutes.

Mix water and arrowroot in a small bowl to come up with a smooth paste.

Pour your arrowroot mixture in the saucepan with the coconut milk mixture. Whisk well to combine, and then bring the mixture to a boil; wait briefly until the mixture begins to shine.

Remove the saucepan from heat, and then slowly mix in the coconut oil using a hand blender. Allow the pot to cool for about 10 minutes.

Once in room temperature, place the pot inside the fridge for about 45 minutes to an hour, until your mixture solidifies and becomes white.

Remove from the fridge; blend once again until fluffy.

Your frosting is now ready to be spread over your cakes and cupcakes.

Banana Ice Cream

Ingredients:

- Coconut oil, 2 tablespoons
- Raw honey, 2 tablespoons
- Ground cinnamon, 1/8 teaspoon
- Peanuts, ½ cup, coarsely chopped
- Pitted dates, 20, roughly chopped
- Vanilla extract, 1 teaspoon
- Bananas, 4 cups, very ripe, sliced
- Cacao nibs, 2 tablespoons

Instructions:

Place dates inside a medium bowl. Cover the bowl with lukewarm water. Set aside to allow dates to soak. After 10 minutes, drain the dates but reserve the soaking liquid.

Use about 3-4 tablespoons of the soaking liquid to puree dates. Mix the soaking liquid with dates with vanilla, cinnamon, coconut oil and honey inside a food processor. Add the ripe bananas, and then puree until the mixture is almost smooth.

Transfer contents into a stainless steel bowl, mix in peanuts and cacao nibs. Cover the bowl and let it freeze. Stir it occasionally until the mixture turns almost solid.

It is recommended to let the banana ice cream soften for a while before serving.

Homemade Deodorant Recipe

Ingredients:

- Coconut oil, 1 ¼ tablespoon
- Beeswax granules, 2 tablespoons
- Shea butter / mango butter / cocoa butter, 1 ¼ tablespoon
- Bentonite clay, ½ tablespoon
- Baking soda / cornstarch / arrowroot, ½ tablespoon
- Rosemary essential oil, 6 drops
- Lemongrass essential oil, 10 drops

Instructions:

Combine beeswax, shea butter, and coconut oil in a double boiler until all ingredients are completely melted and mixed well.

Remove your mixture from heat; pour the mixture into a plastic or glass container. Whisk in your baking soda and bentonite clay until ingredients well combined. Remember that your bentonite clay doesn't match any metal because metals react negatively with it.

Let the mixture sit for a couple of minutes; stir in the essential oils after.

Have a deodorant stick container ready; make sure the plunger is placed all the way down. Pour the mixture carefully into the container.

Allow the mixture to cool and keep the cap off the container until the deodorant has cooled completely. Once cooled, use as normal.

Coconut Hand Scrub

Ingredients:

- Coconut oil, 1 tablespoon
- Raw honey, 2 tablespoons
- Lemon juice, 1 tablespoon
- Sea salt, ¼ cup
- Organic sugar, ¼ cup

Instructions:

In a medium bowl, mix coconut oil and honey together. In a separate bowl, mix sugar, salt and lemon juice until your mixture becomes crumbly.

Pour your salt mixture to your honey mixture and mix them until smooth.

Store the hand scrub inside a small glass container.

To use, just massage a small amount onto your hands for about a minute, rinse your hands with warm water, and then pat dry. You only need to use the scrub once or twice a week.

Coco Lavender Shampoo

Ingredients:

- Coconut oil, 1/3 cup
- Coconut milk, 1/3 cup canned
- Liquid castile soap, 1 cup
- Lavender essential oil, about 50-60 drops

Instructions:

Mix coconut milk and coconut oil together over very low heat. Pour into a clean bottle, and secure the lid. Afterwards, mix the castile soap. Shake the bottle well.

Continue shaking the bottle, and then add the essential oils. (If you don't want lavender, you can use other oils such as peppermint, rosemary, lemongrass or clary sage.) Shake the bottle some more.

The shampoo is now ready to use. Take note, though, that this shampoo is not as thick as the usual commercial shampoos. Squeeze the shampoo directly on your hair. Wash, and then rinse well.

Conclusion

Thank you again for downloading this book!

I hope this book was able to help you realize what a miracle product coconut oil is, what it can be used for, and why it is ideal to have coconut oil inside your home.

The next step is to try some of the steps so you can feel the benefits of coconut oil yourself. Soon, you will be the one singing its praises, and you will end up always making sure that you have a stash of coconut oil at home. With coconut oil, you will look and feel better inside and out. Everyone and everything around you can take advantage of the benefits coconut oil can bring.

Finally, if you enjoyed this book, then I'd like to ask you for a favor, would you be kind enough to leave a review for this book on Amazon? It'd be greatly appreciated!

Thank you and good luck!